1 00

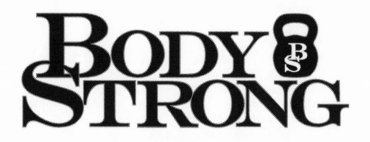

Kettlebell Blitz

BEGINNER PROGRAM

Paul Bova and Robyn Bova

iUniverse, Inc.

New York   Bloomington

iUniverse books may be ordered through booksellers or by contacting:

iUniverse
1663 Liberty Drive
Bloomington, IN 47403
www.iuniverse.com
1-800-Authors (1-800-288-4677)

ISBN: 978-1-4401-1214-0 (soft)
ISBN: 978-1-4401-1215-7 (ebk)

Library of Congress Control Number: 2008911949

Printed in the United States of America

iUniverse rev. date: 12/22/2008

Thank You....

Michael Aron, founder of www.mojotown.com, for your Graphic Consultation. Your vision and insight have made Body Strong a reality.

Sarah Moore of www.writersinthesky.com for editing our book. Your guidance has helped to shape our idea.

Michael Ricca and Tony Antunes, Professional Fitness Equipment Specilaists, for your support and endless supply of Kettlebells.

To our Clients/Friends, for allowing us the opportunity to share what we love with them.

To our Children, for your patience with us through this process. We Love you.

To our Parents, for believing in us and showing us, by example, the joy in teaching and helping others. You have inspired us in more ways than one, and we are forever grateful to all of you.

CONTENTS

ABOUT US

Body Strong, LLC was founded by Paul and Robyn Bova. We created Body Strong because we both have a strong desire to help people attain their fitness goals and live a healthier lifestyle. The programs that we teach to groups and individuals use short duration, higher intensity exercise because we have found, and current research shows, that such an approach is a superior method compared to longer duration, lower intensity activities when the goal is achieving fitness and weight loss. We use mixed modes of exercise combined in constantly varied ways because routine is the enemy of progress when it comes to fitness. The arsenal of tools that we use include; Kettlebells, Sandbags, Resistance Bands, and Bodyweight Exercises.

Our programs are simple yet highly effective, functional and fun, plus they are applicable to anyone. Whether you are new to fitness or a professional athlete, your needs differ by degree, not type. Therefore, at Body Strong, we alter the level of difficulty and not the program. We have found through several years of training our clients that if we were to choose one tool that could, in a single workout, improve cardiovascular health, develop muscular strength, and increase flexibility, it would be the Kettlebell.

We have found with our clients that the Kettlebell has been the tool that has shown the best results in the shortest possible time. While we do not like to say one exercise, or one method, is best, we have found that the Kettlebell comes close to deserving that title.

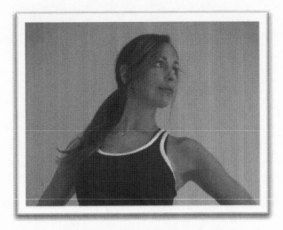

Robyn Bova, AKC

Robyn has been an athlete most of her life. She is certified by the American Kettlebell Club. She started dancing at the age of two and a half. By the time she was sixteen, she was an instructor and went on to co-own and co-direct her own dance studio for twelve years. She worked with children and adults in all areas of dance. During this time, Robyn also was involved with aerobics and weight training. Her passion for fitness grew through these experiences and she decided she wanted to share that energy with others. So, she became a personal trainer and a cardio kickboxing instructor. On a personal level, Robyn learned quickly that spending hours in the gym was not easy for a busy mom of three children, but she knew how important it was to exercise. She believes that "when your body is strong, your mind is clear and your life is better in every aspect." Intense weight training, while effective, can take up a lot of time, make you look and feel bulky, and decrease valuable flexibility that we need especially as we age. Robyn wanted to continue training and, even through battling Lyme Disease, she did so by using Kettlebells. It was an overall workout that did not take a toll on her body and achy joints. In fact, the Kettlebells made her feel stronger and healthier. It slimmed down her entire body and helped to increase her flexibility and mobility with no bulk! Robyn trains clients at the couple's private studio in Stamford, Connecticut.

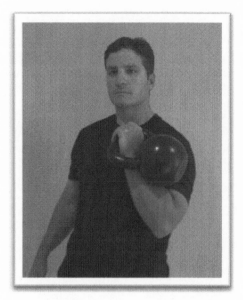

Paul Bova, AKC

Paul has been training clients for over twenty years. He is certified by the American Kettlebell Club. Paul has been active in Martial Arts since the age of eight and Traditional Weight Lifting since he was thirteen. He began fitness instruction in his late teens at his local gym in Connecticut. Paul's love for fitness and its relation to sport began to grow as he started teaching Martial Arts in his late twenties. Paul soon realized that typical weight lifting, while effective, was not the optimal way of training. As a former teacher of Wing Tsun Kung Fu and a current instructor of Commando Krav Maga, Paul began utilizing Kettlebells, Sandbags, and Bodyweight Conditioning in his training program. He found using exercises that were more "functional" helped not only in his Martial Arts performance, but also in his everyday life. Kettlebells became Paul's preferred tool in training as they most closely incorporate real world applications. Today, his respect for Kettlebells has grown not only as a tool for sport, but as a training tool for overall fitness. Paul trains clients at the couple's private studio in Stamford, Connecticut.

ABOUT THE MANUAL

Our program was developed based on experience not only with our clients, but also based on what works for us. We have found that not all Kettlebell exercises are created equal. Meaning that, as a beginner, we feel there are certain exercises with which you should not start[1]. We developed this manual to outline what we call the Kettlebell Blitz Beginner program. The Beginner Program was designed to introduce you to Kettlebells by developing your cardiovascular, muscular strength, and flexibility to allow you to safely advance to our Intermediate and Advanced Programs. This concept will become more apparent as you move up in levels.

All of our programs are designed around being short and intense, hence naming the program "Blitz". Our Beginner program is twenty-five minutes (including the rest periods) and we guarantee that it will be one of the toughest workouts you have ever done. The Body Strong Kettlebell Blitz Beginner program was designed to get your heart rate up quickly and keep it up throughout the entire routine.

If at any point you feel lightheaded or dizzy while doing the routine, you need to put down the Kettlebell. Although this program is a "Beginner" program, it is still difficult to complete, especially if you are new to Kettlebells. As a beginner, the ultimate goal is to be able to get through the entire program while completing all of the exercises with proper form. We will go into more detail on each of these components in the program section of this manual. We do not go by reps, but instead use time as our measure. We have ten (10) two (2)-minute rounds with a thirty (30)-second break in between each round.

- *(1) For example, while we feel the Kettlebell Snatch is a fantastic exercise, it is not something with which we begin our new clients. Rather, we start them out with the Kettlebell High Pull (outlined later in the manual). The High Pull is an excellent transitional exercise to the Snatch. Once you can master the High Pull, which you will in this program, the Snatch, which is introduced in the Intermediate Program, will be an easy transition.*

HISTORY OF KETTLEBELLS

Kettlebells are special weights used to build strength and endurance. Unlike barbells and dumbbells, they look more like a cannon ball with a thick handle attached at the top. Traditional designs are made out of a solid ball of cast iron. Kettlebells come in a variety of sizes with moderate gaps in weights. Some of the lightest Kettlebells measure in at four pounds while the heaviest are 100-plus pounds.

Kettlebell training as we know it today stems from Russia, but there is speculation that Kettlebells were used by Greek athletes and gladiators thousands of years ago. There is also evidence that legendary fighting monks of the famed Shaolin Temple used granite padlocks as a training tool to enhance their kung fu fighting skills. Padlocks are basically a concrete block with a handle on it. The Kettlebells we know today (also known as a handlebell or girya in Russian) has been found in Russian dictionaries dating back to the year 1704. Whether the exact origin of Kettlebells was in Greece, China, or Russia, the history of Kettlebells, as a training tool, dates back over 100 years when they started being used as a form of weight training by strongmen, weightlifters, and wrestlers in Russia. It became a competitive sport in the late 1940s and has progressed in popularity from there.

The Kettlebell has come almost full circle, now being used by fitness enthusiasts, martial artists, and professional athletes, as well as for purposes of rehabilitation. More and more, mainstream health and fitness trainers and clubs are embracing the Kettlebell.

WHY KETTLEBELLS?

Kettlebell training is quickly gaining popularity as the best tool for all-around fitness. The results speak for themselves, but what's unique about a Kettlebell is that it bridges the gap between your cardiovascular training and your weight training. It's the best of both worlds.

Here are a few advantages Kettlebells have over other exercise equipment:

- Natural movement—With Kettlebells, the emphasis is moving the joints in a natural and full range of motion, with equal emphasis on extensor and flexor muscles. The aim with Kettlebells is to develop muscles and joints which can act in the real world through the normal range of motion for the particular muscle or joint.

- All-in-one fitness—Kettlebells give you the advantage of weight training with the flexibility advantages of yoga and the cardiovascular workout of running all in one program. It truly touches all five components of fitness; muscular strength, endurance, flexibility, cardio-respiratory efficiency, and body composition.

- Convenience—Kettlebells are compact and easily transported. Train with them in your house or outside. You even can take them on vacation.

- Enjoyable—The freedom of movement you have, the rhythmic flowing nature of the training itself... it's enjoyable! And let's be honest, an exercise that you do not enjoy is an exercise that you will not do for long.

CHOOSING THE RIGHT KETTLEBELL

Choosing the right Kettlebell is important. Most people new to Kettlebells compare the weight of a Kettlebell to a Dumbbell. Do not compare a Kettlebell pound to a Dumbbell pound. Due to the off-centered design of the Kettlebell, it will recruit and work more muscle fibers during exercises such as the swing, than the balanced nature of a dumbbell weighing the same. We know there are plenty of websites stating the average male should begin with 16kg (35.2 pounds) and the average female should begin with 8kg (17.6 pounds). However, the word "average' means different things to different people.

Before determining the size Kettlebell needed to begin your program, please take into account your overall fitness level, your experience with basic exercises (squat, military press, or chest press), and your degree of flexibility. With that being said, as always, check with your physician before beginning any exercise program.

Experience with our clients has taught us always to start off lightly. We would much rather you learn Kettlebells with a lighter weight first, as it will promote proper form and limit the risk of injury. Believe us, training with a lighter Kettlebell in the beginning stages of your program will definitely get the job done. We suggest being highly comfortable and confident in your form before increasing your weight.

If this is your first time training with Kettlebells, we suggest buying two Kettlebells, one lighter and one heavier. The following is what we recommend to our clients—one 12kg (26.4 pounds) and one 16kg (35.2 pounds) for a male and one 4kg (8.8 pound) and one 8kg (17.6 pound) for a female. Use the smaller Kettlebell to learn proper movements such as the one-arm swing, cleans, and presses. Meanwhile, the heavier Kettlebell would be great for your squat and lunge movements, two-handed swings, and one-arm rows.

BASIC SAFETY PRECAUTIONS

Before you begin make sure that you take the following safety precautions (You will find a detailed description of each in the Guidelines and Safety section):

- Always train somewhere you will be able to drop your Kettlebell if it becomes necessary.

- Always stay focused. Kettlebell training needs 100% attention at all times. You should not train while watching TV, reading, etc.

- You should train either barefoot or in flat-soled shoes. Typical running shoes have an elevated heel and can make it difficult to maintain proper form, as you have to load your weight into the heels.

- Never train with the sunlight, or any light, directly in your eyes

- Pay attention to your surroundings; make sure that you have enough room to execute the exercises safely.

- Build up to heavier weight gradually.

- Do not allow the Kettlebell to bang against your forearm during the performance of any exercise.

- Always keep your head straight or facing up. Never tuck your chin into your body as it can put strain on your neck.

- Use proper breathing.

- Always keep proper Kettlebell form throughout all of the exercises.

EXERCISES

The following pages are a step-by-step guide showing the exercises we will use in our Body Strong Kettlebell Blitz Beginner program. We suggest reading through each of the exercises and reviewing the illustrations. With your lighter Kettlebell, practice each of the movements until you feel comfortable. You should only begin the program once you feel as though you can safely execute each exercise.

The following are some basics with which you should acquaint yourself with before picking up the bell.

Proper Kettlebell Breathing: As a general rule of thumb, when the Kettlebell is coming towards you breathe in, when going away breathe out. You should never exhale all of your breath, as blowing out all of your air will relax the body too much and make it difficult and unsafe to hold the Kettlebell.

Proper Kettlebell Alignment: Stand with your feet shoulder-width apart. Your toes should be pointed forward. Lean your weight back into your heels. A good way to check if your weight is in your heels is to wiggle your toes. Squat back as if you were going to sit in a chair. Your knees should be in line with your hips and not reaching over past your toes. Squeeze your glutes to take the strain off your knees. Hold a slight curve in your back. Without arching, focus on pulling your stomach into your spine and relaxing your back. Pull your shoulders down and back. You are now in proper Kettlebell alignment.

Kettlebell Grip: When gripping the bell, you want to be sure that you loosen your grip at the pinky while keeping most of the grip power in your thumb, index, and middle fingers.

KETTLEBELL SWINGS

Swing: The Swing is one of the foundational exercises in Kettlebell training. The proper hip thrust necessary for swings will apply to many other Kettlebell exercises. Swings teach you how to generate power from the feet up through the body. This exercise is great at developing your hamstrings, calves, shoulders and glutes. Place one Kettlebell between your feet, with your legs about shoulder width apart. While pushing your backside out, bend your knees to get into the starting position. Make sure that your back is flat and look straight ahead. Grab the Kettlebell with two hands while looking straight ahead. Swing the Kettlebell back between your legs. Quickly reverse the direction and drive through with your hips taking the Kettlebell straight out in front of you. The proper motion involves locking your knees and contracting your glutes in order to snap the hip. You should be pushing hard against the ground as you straighten your legs. Let the Kettlebell swing back between your legs and repeat. A good way to think about the swing is that your body is like a spring. You are loading your body like a spring and then exploding with your legs pushing off the ground, locking your knees and snapping your hips forward as you tighten your glutes. Inhale on the swing between your legs and exhale when you raise the Kettlebell.

The one-handed swings are the same as the two-handed exercise without the second hand on the bell. One-handed swings are not much more difficult than two-handed swings since the swing in general relies heavily on the explosive power you generate from driving up with your legs and snapping with your knees and hips.

Switching between hands takes coordination, but is easily mastered once the proper swing form is developed. At the top of your swing you will notice when switching hands that the bell will almost float for a split second allowing you time to grab it in midair.

Two-Handed Swing - Front View

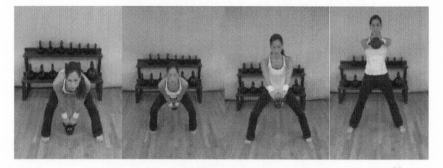

One-Handed Swing – Front View

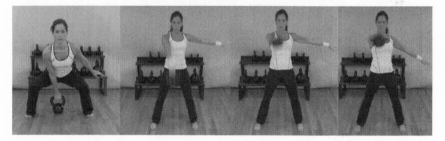

Two-Handed Swing – Side View

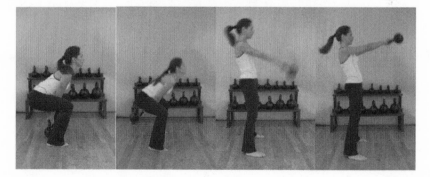

HALO & GOOD MORNING

Halo: This is a great exercise to develop shoulder mobility. Get the Kettlebell into the bottom up position (shown in the photo) in front of your face. In one smooth motion make a circle around the head while keeping the Kettlebell as low and as tight to your body as you can. Make sure that you do not arch your back while performing the Halo. A good way to prevent an arched back is to squeeze your thighs and glutes. This exercise should be done slowly, reversing the movement each cycle (once to the left and then once to the right).

Good Morning: This is one of the best exercises to develop your lower back, glutes, and hamstrings. Begin by placing the bell on your back; in about the same position as you would a squat. The first thing to move during a good morning should be your hips. With a very slight bend in your knees, push your hips back and begin the descent. A good way to think about the movement is that your backside is being pulled towards the wall. You should maintain a good arch in your lower back and keep your head up. Continue until your back is about parallel to the floor and then raise yourself back up. You can use a wide, medium, or close stance when doing a good morning. Like the Halo, you should perform this exercise slowly.

Halo

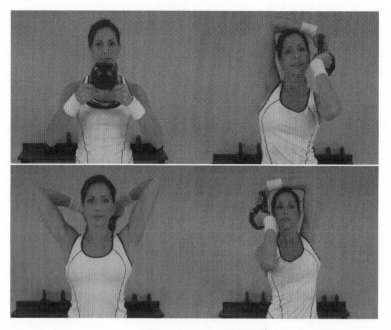

Good Morning

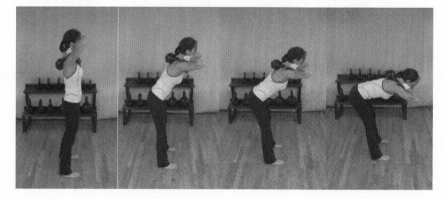

DEAD CLEAN & PRESS

Dead Clean: The clean is another foundational exercise in the Kettlebell program. This exercise works the hamstrings, lower back, and traps. The clean is a way to bring the Kettlebell to your shoulder. Stand over the Kettlebell with your feet placed slightly wider than shoulder-width apart. Make sure the Kettlebell is centered between your legs (please remember proper Kettlebell alignment). Squat down slowly and grab the handle of the Kettlebell with one hand and allow your other arm to rest at your side in a neutral position. Stand up in the motion of a dead lift, being sure to keep your back straight. Drive up with your hips sending the Kettlebell up instead of forward (like in a swing). Pull your arm close to your body and turn your palm toward your body as you send the Kettlebell up toward your shoulder. Punch through at the end (do not curl the Kettlebell). Bend your elbow completely; ending with the back of your thumb facing your upper chest and your elbow should be down on or toward the hip bone. The Kettlebell should be resting comfortably between the "V" made by your upper and lower arm (this is called the "Rack" position). When performing the clean the Kettlebell should not slam into your forearm; rather it should roll around your arm at the top of the movement. Continue to practice until you have a smooth Clean.

Press: This exercise mainly works the shoulders and triceps. From the "Rack" position and looking straight ahead, press the Kettlebell out and overhead as if you are trying to make half of a circle. Continue to press the Kettlebell behind your head and lean forward slightly at the top for a stronger lockout. Get the weight to a fully raised position with your elbow locked, making sure that you do not extend your shoulder. Keep it there for one second. Lower the Kettlebell back to the Rack position.

Dead Clean & Press – Front View

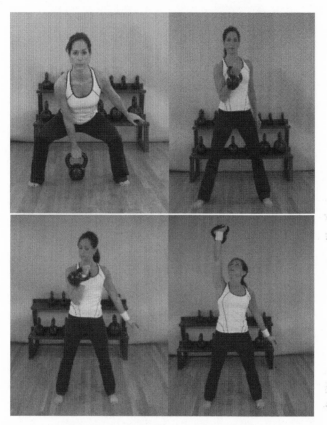

Dead Clean & Press – Side View

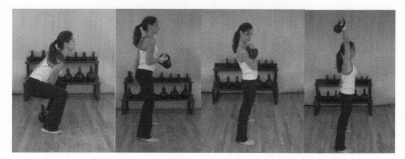

AROUND THE BODY PASS
& ONE-ARM ROW

Around the Body Pass: This exercise is a great core workout that also develops grip and shoulder strength. Pick up the Kettlebell and hold it with both hands loosely at your waist. Your palms should be facing in towards your body. Throughout the exercise, you should keep your back straight and your toes pointed forward. Protect your lower back and work your core by keeping your abdominal muscles engaged at all times. Your shoulders should be down and back in a relaxed position throughout the entire exercise. Swing the Kettlebell around your right side, releasing your left hand and bringing your left arm around to your back. Switch hands on the handle of the Kettlebell when it reaches your back and bring it around to the front with your left hand. Switch again at the front of your body, and continue the slingshot motion around your waist. The key to this exercise is to maintain a tight core and breathe throughout the movement.

One-Arm Row: The one-arm Kettlebell row is a great exercise to work on the lats and biceps. Using the example of the left arm, here is how you do a one-arm Kettlebell row. Place a Kettlebell next to the inside of your right foot. Place your left foot behind your back and rest your right elbow on your right leg. Pull the Kettlebell off of the floor to your stomach. Keep your back flat at all times and your head facing forward. You may vary the movement by adding a twisting motion to your grip as you raise the Kettlebell upward.

Around the Body Pass

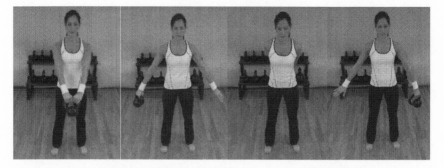

One-Arm Kettlebell Row – Front View

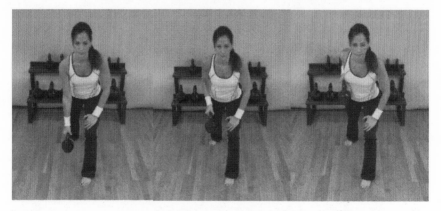

One-Arm Kettlebell Row – Side View

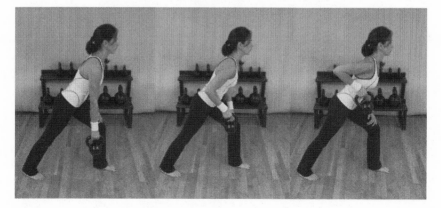

ONE-ARM CHEST PRESS

One-Arm Chest Press: This exercise is similar to the standard bench press and is great for strengthening the chest and tricep muscles. Lie on the floor and position the Kettlebell for one arm to press. The arm being worked should be out at 90 degrees to the torso and the forearm 90 degrees to the upper part of your arm (Please be sure to keep your wrist straight during this exercise). While pressing your lower back into the floor, squeeze the bell hard and straighten your arm. The bell will now be hanging almost overhead. Slowly return the bell to the starting position. Imagine that you are trying to push yourself through the floor for added stability and increased strength.

Please be careful when performing this exercise not to become too fatigued, as your arm could give way and cause the Kettlebell to land on top of you. If you feel as if you cannot complete the full minute on each side, it is acceptable to switch sides every ten or fifteen seconds (When switching arms, remember to pass the Kettlebell over your stomach, not your face). The ultimate goal is to reach a minute on each side safely. Please use your best judgment when performing any exercise which has the Kettlebell positioned over your body.

One-Arm Chest Press – Side View

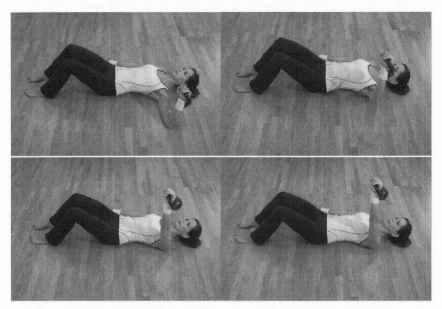

One-Arm Chest Press - Rear View

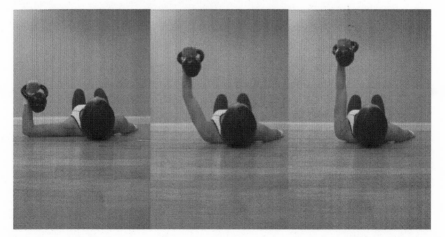

WINDMILL & OVERHEAD SQUAT

Windmill: This exercise mainly works the oblique muscles and hamstrings, as well as strengthens your shoulders. Begin by cleaning and pressing a Kettlebell overhead with one arm. Your arm will remain locked throughout the entire movement. Push your hip out in the direction of the locked-out Kettlebell. Turn your feet out at a forty-five degree angle from the arm with the Kettlebell. Keep your eyes on the Kettlebell at all times. Lower yourself until you can touch the floor in the opposite direction (if you cannot touch the floor, try to go down as far as possible). Pause for a second and then reverse the motion back to the starting position. Remember to keep your rear leg locked; your front leg should remain locked as well, however it can bend slightly. The Windmill should be performed slowly and with great control.

Overhead Squat: The overhead squat is great for your quadriceps, hamstrings and glutes, as well as a superb shoulder stretch and strengthener. Clean and press a Kettlebell overhead with one arm[2]. Your arm will remain locked throughout the entire movement. Keep your eyes on the Kettlebell at all times. Push your backside out and squat as low as possible. While lowering into the squat, place your hand without the Kettlebell on the floor. Pause at the bottom position for a second before rising back to the top.

Note: Both the Windmill and Overhead Squat require the Kettlebell to be over your body. Please be careful when performing this exercise not to become too fatigued as your arm could give way.

-    *(2) In the Kettlebell Beginner Blitz program, you will be alternating between Windmills and Overhead Squats, so the Kettlebell will already be in the overhead position after you complete the Windmill*

Windmill

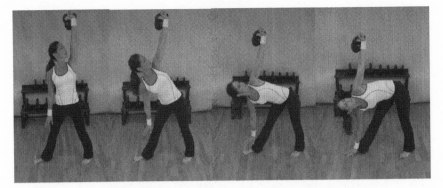

Overhead Squat – Front View

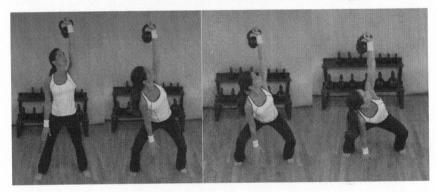

Overhead Squat – Side View

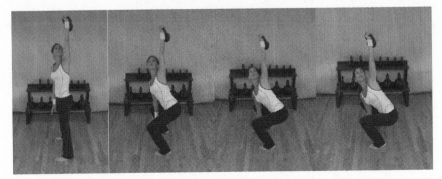

LUNGES & SUMO ROWS

Lunges: This exercise is great for working the glutes, quadriceps and calves. Hold the Kettlebell firmly in your right hand in the "rack" position. Stand up straight with your feet about hip width apart. Maintain proper body posture as you step your left leg back as far as possible, bending your front knee so that it is at a 90 degree angle (Be sure that your knee does not extend beyond your toes). Shift your center of gravity to the mid-point of the body; raise your heel on your rear leg ensuring that the ball of your foot is in contact with the ground. Lower your body to the floor by dropping your back knee (Imagine the back knee dropping in a line vertically downward). Bring your rear knee as close to the floor as you can without touching the floor. Immediately raise back up again without locking out your back leg and repeat. Note that you will do this exercise continually on one side for 30 seconds in the Beginner program.

Sumo Rows: This exercise is great for working the glutes, hamstrings, and calves as well as the shoulders. Stand with your legs apart and your toes pointed outward. Your feet should be wider than hip distance apart so that when you squat down your knees stay out over your toes and do not turn inward. Your Kettlebell should be on the ground in between your feet. Keeping your back flat, squat all the way down to the floor by bending your knees. Grab the handle of your Kettlebell with both hands. Use your legs to stand up quickly into an upright position. As you push to standing, pull the Kettlebell upward until it is at chin level. At the top of the exercise, you should be standing straight up with the Kettlebell at your chin and your elbows pointing up and out. This is one quick movement using all of your muscles to push your body up while simultaneously pulling the Kettlebell up to your chin. Lower the Kettlebell all the way back down to the ground, squatting with your legs until the Kettlebell touches the floor.

Lunge

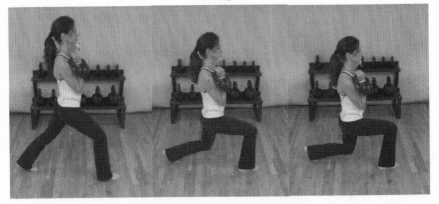

Sumo Row – Front View

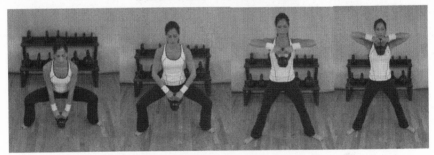

Sumo Row – Side View

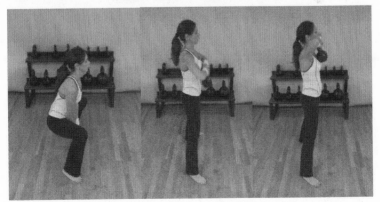

BI-TRI COMBO

Bi-Tri Combo: This exercise is great for building your biceps and triceps as well as your shoulders. Begin by wrapping your hands around the Kettlebell. The Kettlebell should be positioned at about waist height with your arms extended in front of your body (as shown in the photo). With your head straight, begin to curl the weight up to your shoulders. Your thumbs should almost be touching your chest. At the top of the motion, press the Kettlebell overhead (You may have to move your head back slightly to press the Kettlebell above your head, however, be careful not to drop your chin down). At the top of the press, begin slowly to lower the Kettlebell down, by bending your elbows, until the handle touches the back of your neck. Extend your arms back over your head and lower the bell down to your chest. Slowly lower the weight back to the starting position and repeat. This exercise should be performed slowly with no body movement. If you find yourself swaying your body to curl the weight, then you should lower the weight you are using. Remember to keep proper form throughout the entire routine.

During the Body Strong Kettlebell Blitz Beginner Program you will be asked to isolate your biceps and triceps while doing this exercise. You will perform this exercise as described above as well as perform 30 seconds of just triceps extensions and 30 seconds of just bicep curls.

Note: The Bi-Tri Combo requires the Kettlebell to be over your body. Please be careful when performing this exercise not to become too fatigued as your arms could give way.

Bi-Tri Combo - Front View

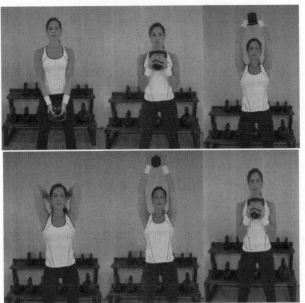

Bi-Tri Combo – Side View

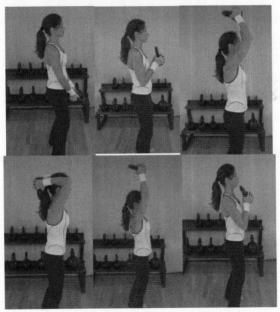

HIGH PULL

High Pull: This exercise is great for working the shoulders, back and hamstrings. The Kettlebell High Pull is an excellent exercise in itself. However, we use it primarily as a transition for the Kettlebell Snatch, which you will learn in the Intermediate program.

Similar to the Swing, place one Kettlebell between your feet, with your legs about shoulder width apart. While pushing your backside out, bend your knees to get into the starting position. Make sure that your back is flat and look straight ahead. Grab the Kettlebell with one hand while looking straight ahead. Swing the Kettlebell back between your legs. Quickly reverse the direction and drive through with your hips taking the Kettlebell straight out in front of you. The proper motion involves locking your knees and contracting your glutes in order to snap the hip. You should be pushing hard against the ground as you straighten your legs. Lift the Kettlebell until it is slightly above shoulder level. Once in this position pull the Kettlebell back, towards your body, by bending the elbow slightly. The Kettlebell will be positioned around eye level and should form an extension of your forearm. Your arm and the Kettlebell should be parallel with the ground at the top of the movement. Lean into the Kettlebell the moment you are finishing the pull, and then quickly punch the Kettlebell forward again and let it swing down between your legs.

Repeat the high pull by allowing the Kettlebell to fall as you squat once again. This time, allow the Kettlebell to swing between your legs and then lift once again.

High Pull – Front View

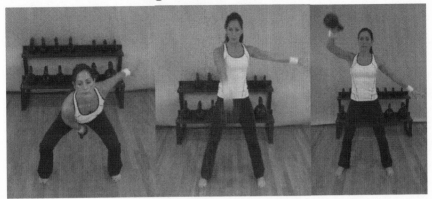

High Pull – Side View

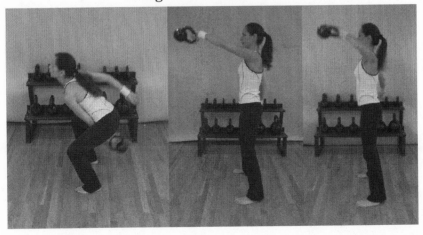

KB CRUNCH & RUSSIAN TWIST

KB Crunch: This exercise is not only great for your abdominals, but it also works the chest and triceps. Lie with your back on the floor (or mat) with your feet flat on the ground and your knees bent. Begin by simultaneously raising your torso in a crunching fashion and pressing the Kettlebell to an overhead position. Raise your torso up until your back is completely off of the floor and your hands are stretched out toward your knees, locking your elbows. Slowly lower down to the original start position and repeat. Remember to squeeze your abs tight throughout the motion. If this exercise becomes difficult with the Kettlebell in your hand, safely place the Kettlebell on the floor and continue with no weight.

Russian Twist: This exercise develops core strength, rotational power, and dynamic stability. Sit with your knees bent and your heels on the floor. Hold the Kettlebell by the handle (bottom down) in the center of your body. Begin to rotate the bell slowly from side to side with your head following the Kettlebell at all times. To start, keep your triceps against your torso as you do the movement. As you gain strength, move the Kettlebell farther away from your body.

KB Crunch

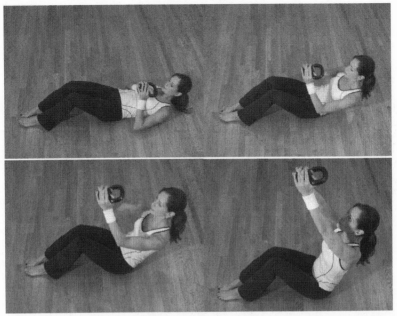

Russian Twist

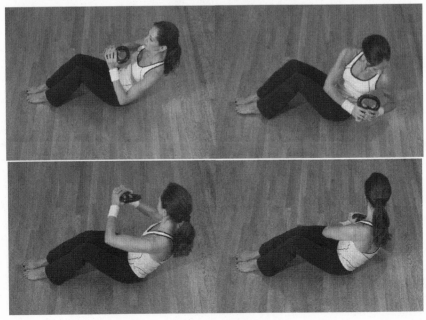

BODY STRONG KETTLEBELL BLITZ BEGINNER PROGRAM

Now that you understand the Kettlebell exercises, it is time for the program. We use this program three times a week with our clients and all have shown significant gains in muscular strength, endurance, flexibility, cardio-respiratory efficiency, and body composition. The Body Strong Blitz Beginner Program focuses on minimum rest and maximum muscle exhaustion.

Instead of using reps, we go by time. We found that by using time as our goal, our clients do not have to count reps and they just can focus on their form. We also found that long, paced, high rep sets have a dramatic effect on tendon and ligament strength. Over-developed muscles without adequate tendon strength can lead to overload and injury. High repetition sets help to strengthen the tendons and ligaments.

Our program is designed to build you up to our Intermediate and Advanced programs. We want to strengthen your muscles first before you attempt more difficult exercises. If you are having difficulty completing a set, our first suggestion is to try to rest with the Kettlebell in your hand (i.e. if you are doing an overhead squat, rest with the Kettlebell in the fully locked position above your head). However, if you are feeling lightheaded or dizzy, put the Kettlebell down. You have plenty of time to complete the program; there is no reason to rush your development. It is always better to be safe than sorry.

You will need two things to complete this program - a Kettlebell and a clock or interval timer. When reviewing the exercises, please refer back to the book and practice each exercise before attempting to go through the program. Or, visit our website www.bodystrong.org to view each exercise in slow motion and in real time.

Remember, Form! Form! Form! - Do not cheat your way to completing this program; make sure that you are using proper form. If you feel like you are doing an exercise incorrectly or something does not feel right, <u>STOP</u> immediately. Only you know your own body and limitations. Please make sure that you listen to your body. If you feel like you are pushing yourself too hard, stop the exercise. There is plenty of time to complete this program. However, if you push yourself too hard in the beginning you could be faced with an injury that will set back your training for weeks. Be smart about your training and slowly build up your programs.

With that being said, the way we train a majority of our new clients is to begin this program with one-minute rounds and ninety seconds of rest. If you decide to alter the program to one-minute rounds, be sure that you also alter the switches we have outlined in the program to match your time (i.e., 30 seconds will become 15 seconds and one minute will become 30 seconds). The following is an altered one-minute Swing Routine with a 90-second rest:

SWINGS	
Time	**Exercises / Side**
15 Seconds	Two-Handed Swing
15 Seconds	Left-Hand Swing
15 Seconds	Right-Hand Swing
15 Seconds	Hand-to-Hand Swing
Rest – 90 Seconds	

Your goal is to continue this program until you can successfully execute each exercise for the full two minutes with only a thirty-second rest period between each one.

The following pages will outline the Body Strong Kettlebell Blitz Beginner Program. We suggest that you write down or photocopy the program so it is readily accessible while you are doing the routine.

KETTLEBELL SWINGS	
Time	**Exercises / Side**
30 Seconds	Two-Handed Swing
30 Seconds	Left-Hand Swing
30 Seconds	Right-Hand Swing
30 Seconds	Hand-to-Hand Swing
Rest – 30 Seconds	

HALO & GOOD MORNING	
Time	**Exercises / Side**
30 Seconds	Halo
30 Seconds	Good Morning
30 Seconds	Halo
30 Seconds	Good Morning
Rest – 30 Seconds	

DEAD CLEAN & PRESS	
Time	**Execsises / Side**
1 Minute	Left
1 Minute	Right
Rest – 30 Seconds	

AROUND THE BODY & ONE-ARM ROW	
Time	**Exercises / Side**
30 Seconds	Around the Body - Right
30 Seconds	One Arm Rows - Right
30 Seconds	Around the Body - Left
30 Seconds	One Arm Rows - Left
Rest – 30 Seconds	

ONE-ARM CHEST PRESS	
Time	**Exercises / Side**
1 Minute	Left
1 Minute	Right
Rest – 30 Seconds	

WINDMILL & OVERHEAD SQUAT	
Time	**Exercises / Side**
1 Minute	Left
1 Minute	Right
Rest – 30 Seconds	

LUNGES & SUMO ROWS	
Time	**Exercises / Side**
30 Seconds	Lunges - Right
30 Seconds	Sumo Rows
30 Seconds	Lunges - Left
30 Seconds	Sumo Rows
Rest – 30 Seconds	

BI-TRI COMBO	
Time	**Exercises / Side**
30 Seconds	Full Range
30 Seconds	Tricep Extension
30 Seconds	Bicep Curl
30 Seconds	Full Range
Rest – 30 Seconds	

HIGH PULL	
Time	**Exercises / Side**
1 Minute	Left
1 Minute	Right
Rest – 30 Seconds	

KB CRUNCH & RUSSIAN TWIST	
Time	**Exercises / Side**
30 Seconds	KB Crunch
30 Seconds	Russian Twist
30 Seconds	KB Crunch
30 Seconds	Russian Twist
Rest – 30 Seconds	

CONGRATULATIONS!

If you made it through the program without having to put the Kettlebell down, well done! If you needed to take some breaks in between exercises, don't be discouraged. Continue the program three times a week, resting a day in between workouts until you can complete the entire program as outlined. Once you get comfortable with the program, try to speed up each set. While we do not encourage counting reps, in a typical two-minute swing cycle we will perform over eighty reps. If you find yourself having an easy time with this program in a couple of weeks, work on increasing your speed or repetitions in the time allotted.

Another way to increase the intensity of your workout is to increase the weight you are using, always being aware of your form. We find with our clients that by increasing the weight of their Kettlebell, they will feel like beginners all over again with any exercise they are performing.

One final way to increase the intensity of the program is to institute an "active rest." An active rest period is when you stay physically active during the thirty-second rest breaks. You can choose to do Jumping Jacks, Burpies, Run in Place … anything to keep your heart rate up.

We hope you enjoy the Body Strong Kettlebell Blitz Beginner Program. We look forward to your success with Kettlebells.

We are always available to answer questions. Please email us at info@bodystrong.org.

Sincerely,
Paul & Robyn Bova

GUIDELINES AND SAFETY

One of our mottos at Body Strong is "Safety First." Safety does not only pertain to correct form--it also includes being aware of your surroundings as well as knowing your limitations. The following are guidelines and safety rules with which anyone starting a Kettlebell routine should become familiar:

Always train somewhere you will be able to drop your Kettlebell if you get into trouble. Make sure that you have enough room to execute the exercises safely without harming other people, objects, or yourself. Being aware of your surroundings is important. If you lose your Kettlebell while training, you want to be sure that it is not going to break anything or, worse, harm someone. The Kettlebell is made of cast iron. Make sure there is enough space between you and any training partners at all times.

Always stay focused. Kettlebell training needs 100% attention at all times. You should not train while watching television shows, reading, etc. You also should never train with the sunlight, or any light, directly in your eyes. Having the sun in your eyes either from direct sunlight, from sun glare off windows or mirrors, or other direct lighting can be distracting and cause you to lose focus.

Train in Bare Feet or Flat Soled Shoes. You should train either barefoot or in flat-soled shoes. Typical running shoes have an elevated heel and can make it difficult to maintain proper form as you have to load your weight into the heels. Sneakers might feel comfortable, but they can throw off your body alignment as well as cause you to lose contact with the ground. You should also make sure that you always train on a flat surface

Use proper breathing. As a general rule of thumb, when the Kettlebell is coming towards you breathe in, when going away breath out. You should never exhale all of your breath, as blowing out all of your air will relax the body too much and make it difficult and unsafe to hold the Kettlebell. In addition to proper breathing, be sure when beginning the program not to stop moving when you finish an exercise, especially if you are winded or your heart is beating hard. If you stop moving, your blood pressure will spike and that can be harmful. Instead of standing still or sitting down, keep your body moving. Walk around the room or walk in place until your breath and heart rate return to normal.

Build up to heavier weight gradually. The size and weight of the Kettlebell is not that important. What is important is using the correct form, emphasis, and focus of the body as well as expression of the technique. If you cannot perform the techniques with a light Kettlebell with solid form, then why try a heavier bell? Your form will not improve and you are at risk of injuring yourself. This is not traditional weight lifting. You need to move away from the mentality that the more weight you can lift, the stronger you are. There is a time when you will want to use heavier Kettlebells. This should be after the form of whatever you are performing is correct and after you can handle the current weight you are using. Again, keep in mind the size of the Kettlebell is not as important as perfection of the form.

Do not go to failure. Many people who lift weights or train in other disciplines believe in going to the point of muscle failure. We strongly suggest against this approach. There is no need to go to failure when training with the Kettlebell. Think about this. You are performing an over head press. You start to fail. The weight of the bells can come crashing down on you, or you might drop the weight with your hands gripped in the handle and end up hurting your back. It is not worth it. Trust us. You will be able to build up your conditioning, strength, and endurance without putting yourself in a possibly dangerous situation.

Do not try and catch the Kettlebell if you lose it during an exercise. Instead of trying to catch or stop the Kettlebell, get out of its way and let it fall, or guide it down to the ground. The worst that can happen is you damage the floor or the Kettlebell itself.

Do not allow the Kettlebell to bang against your forearm during the performance of any exercise. Make sure that when you are doing the clean, the Kettlebell is rotating around your arm and not coming over your hand. Follow the guidelines in this book and practice, practice, practice!

Always keep your head straight or facing up. Never tuck your chin into your body as it can put strain on your neck. Keep the neck neutral-aligned, not too far forward or backward. There is a tendency not to move the head with the trunk of the body but instead keep the head up and facing forward. This typically happens when dead lifting the Kettlebell off the floor or at the bottom of a swing. Instead of looking forward, keep the head in line with the body. At the bottom of a swing, you will be looking down at the corner of the floor ahead of you. Also, be careful not to dip your head down when looking down, as this will pitch your head too far forward and cause neck strain.

Move your hips first, while keeping your arms loose. Moving your hips first on a clean, swing or high pull is safest for your back and knees. Drive with your glutes and hamstrings, less with your quads, and not at all with your back or your arms. During the movement make sure your arms stay loose. Should your arms tense up, especially on a downswing, you could risk injuring your elbows.

Brace your Abdominals. Protect your back by keeping your abdominal muscles contracted. To correctly brace, you should attempt to pull your navel back in toward your spine. Be careful not to hold your breath; you should be able to breathe evenly while bracing.

Always start each exercise in Proper Kettlebell Alignment. Lean your weight back into your heels. Wiggle your toes to check if all of your weight is back on your heels. Squat back as if you were going to sit in a chair. Your knees should be in line with your hips and not reaching over past your toes. Squeeze your glutes to take the strain off your knees. Hold a slight curve in your back. Without arching, focus on pulling your stomach into your spine and relaxing your back. Do not round your lower back when picking the Kettlebell up or when putting it down.

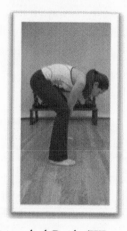

Rounded Back (Wrong)

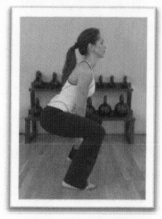

Curved Back (Right)

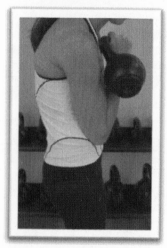

Rounded Back (Wrong)

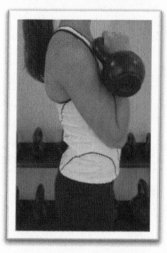

Curved Back (Right)

Pull your shoulders down and back. This concept is an important part of maintaining proper Kettlebell alignment. You can avoid straining your neck and back by keeping your shoulders in the right position. Proper technique also protects the shoulders and puts most of the work on the scapula and the lats.

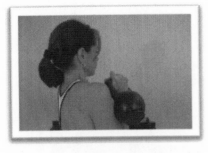 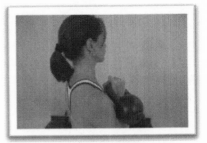

Shoulders Hunched (Wrong)   Shoulders Down & Back (Right)

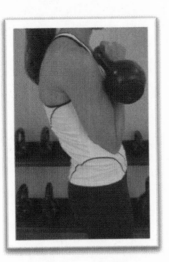 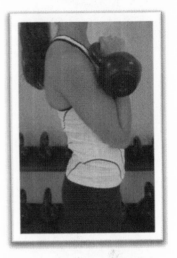

Shoulders Rounded (Wrong)   Down & Back (Right)

Don't overextend your shoulders. Make sure that you do not overextend your shoulder in the front plane when moving your arms over your chest. This requirement holds true when doing floor presses, bench presses, pushups, etc. Also, do not extend the shoulders out of your down and back position when pressing the Kettlebell overhead. Overextending your shoulders is dangerous and you are only opening yourself up to injury.

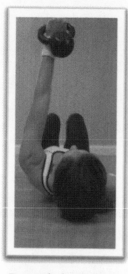

Extended (Wrong)

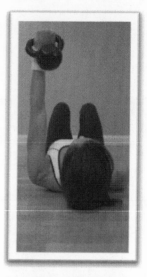

Not Extended (Right)

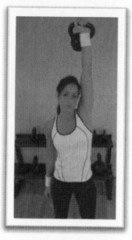

Extended (Wrong)

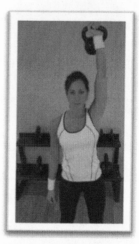

Not Extended (Right)

Keep your wrists straight, do not bend them. There are a handful of techniques for which you do bend your wrist, but for the majority of the techniques this is not the case. Your wrist should be straight and not bent at any point of the technique.

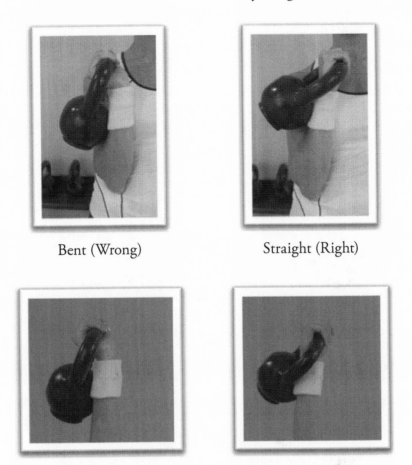

Bent (Wrong)   Straight (Right)

Bent (Wrong)   Straight (Right)

It is impossible to cover every situation when it comes to safety. You need to rely on your own common sense. The most important thing is to have fun. Kettlebell training, while intense, is a lot of fun to perform. It is unlike any other training program around. Enjoy yourself and be safe!

Made in the USA
Lexington, KY
02 October 2010